IO104498

Table of Contents

"Betrayal may wound the heart, but only bitterness can corrupt the assignment. Stay postured in purity."

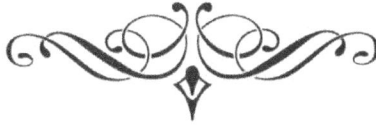

Chapter One

The Reality of Betrayal in Leadership

"Yea, mine own familiar friend, in whom I trusted, which did eat of my bread, hath lifted up his heel against me."
Psalm 41:9 (KJV)

As we endeavor to build in natural or spiritual professions, there are always people who don't stay the course. A significant leadership challenge that arises while working to build healthy organizations is betrayal. Betrayal brings adverse consequences and often causes setbacks from prior progress and accomplishment.

Betrayal has several working definitions:

- Failing to meet declared expectations in a covenant relationship.
- Deserting your post, position, or responsibilities prematurely.

- Violating confidence placed in an individual or relationship.

As leaders engage with other leaders, staff, and volunteers in the context of building healthy businesses, ministries, and community organizations, it's important to be able to trust those that you work with in a consistent manner.

In Scripture, trust is tied to fruit.

"A faithful man shall abound with blessings: but he that maketh haste to be rich shall not be innocent. *"Proverbs 28:20 (KJV)*

The quality of being trustworthy as team members is paramount to building healthy organizations. No one wants to engage in a dysfunctional organization for very long. The need for organizational health highlights the need for devotion, commitment, and loyalty in key relationships.

Devotion and loyalty are not merely emotional traits—they are Kingdom characteristics.

"And the things that thou hast heard of me among many witnesses, the same commit thou to faithful men, who shall be able to teach others also."*2 Timothy 2:2 (KJV)*

HANDLING BETRAYAL

BETRAYAL

WITH GRACE

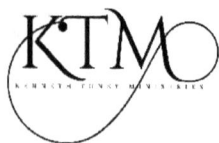
KENNETH TONG MINISTRIES

Handling Betrayal with Grace

Copyright © 2025 Kenneth E. Toney

All rights reserved. No portion of this book may be reproduced, stored in a retrieval system, or transmitted in any form or by any means—electronic, mechanical, photocopying, recording, or otherwise—without the prior written permission of the author. Brief quotations may be used in literary reviews and academic discussions.

Unless otherwise noted, Scripture quotations marked (KJV) are taken from The Holy Bible, King James Version (Public Domain).
Scripture quotations marked (AMP) are taken from The Amplified Bible, Copyright © 1954, 1958, 1962, 1964, 1965, 1987 by The Lockman Foundation. Used by permission. All rights reserved.

Scripture quotations marked (ESV) are from The Holy Bible, English Standard Version, Copyright © 2001 by Crossway, a publishing ministry of Good News Publishers. Used by permission. All rights reserved.
Scripture quotations marked (NLT) are taken from The Holy Bible, New Living Translation, Copyright © 1996, 2004, 2007 by Tyndale House Foundation. Used by permission. All rights reserved.

ISBN: 979-8-218-81263-8
First Edition: 2025

Published by: Kenneth E. Toney
Edited by: Creative Concepts for Ministry
Cover Art by: Creative Concepts for Ministry
Elevation & Development by: Creative Concepts for Ministry
Consultant: Apostle Connie A. Dotson
Email: creativeconcepts4ministry@gmail.com

Contact Information:
Ken Toney Ministries – ktmonline.org
Dwelling Place Int'l Church – dpicalive.org
Email: apostleken@dpicalive.org

Mailing Address:
Dwelling Place Int'l Church C/O Ken Toney
114 East Highway 72 Collierville, TN 38017

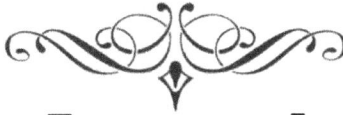

Foreword

Apostle Stephen A. Garner

Lead Pastor Rivers Chicago Illinois

There are subjects and topics that need to be discussed on a regular basis. The subject of betrayal is one of them. Most people would rather not discuss it. I believe this is due in part to the perceived trauma betrayal has imposed upon the whole of humanity.

Satan himself betrayed God because of his pride and lost his place in Gods realm. He was banished to the earth. I personally believe he's spinned a web like a spider over the landscape of humanity called betrayal.

The desecration of covenant relationships, a willful neglect of one's duties or intentional withdrawal from deeds that empower others are all forms of betrayal. There's no pretty or decent end to betrayal. Its goal is to mar people and leave them drowning in pools of bitterness and regret.

Apostle Ken Toney, inspired by God has created a strategy and template to overcome the deadly webs of betrayal. This booklet is a blueprint to help the reader identify betrayal. There's also a practical approach on how to disarm it in your life.

The spirit of betrayal comes to undermine organizational health by eroding devotion, commitment, and loyalty in key relationships.

This is not just an emotional disturbance—it is a spiritual breach.

"Every kingdom divided against itself is brought to desolation; and every city or house divided against itself shall not stand." *Matthew 12:25 (KJV)*

We see a breakdown in a key relationship that caused significant harm to the ministry and life of Jesus as He is betrayed by His trusted disciple Judas Iscariot. Judas held a position of trust as the treasurer of Jesus' traveling evangelistic ministry. Unfortunately, the spirit of betrayal often enters our most trusted co-laborers, advisors, and friends.

John 13:2–11 (KJV) *"And supper being ended, the devil having now put into the heart of Judas Iscariot, Simon's son, to betray him;*
Jesus knowing that the Father had given all things into his hands, and that he was come from God, and went to God; He riseth from supper, and laid aside his garments; and took a towel, and girded himself...For he knew who should betray him; therefore said he, Ye are not all clean."

Even in betrayal, Jesus remained in posture. He washed Judas' feet, showing us, that leadership doesn't lose its integrity even when surrounded by disloyalty. This teaches us that true leaders don't retaliate—they respond with humility and honor, even when dishonor is present.

As we know from studying scripture, we knew that Jesus being betrayed by Judas was necessary for the fulness of Christ's assignment in the earth to be accomplished.

There are betrayals that break us, but there are also betrayals that build us.

"That thou doest, do quickly." *John 13:27 (KJV)* Jesus did not try to prevent the betrayal—He discerned its purpose. He understood that betrayal often ushers us into fulfillment if we remain postured before the Father.

Notice that the devil himself injected a thought into the heart of Judas Iscariot to betray Jesus. Jesus continues to wash the feet of the Disciples including Judas, knowing that the time of His betrayal had come and that it would be at the hand of a very close friend.

The enemy doesn't always destroy from the outside—he injects thoughts into those closest to us.

"The thief cometh not, but for to steal, and to kill, and to destroy..." *John 10:10 (KJV)*

As leaders, we must not only guard our own hearts but teach those around us how to guard theirs, lest the enemy find access through the open door of offense, pride, or ambition.

As leaders, we have to be aware that the spirit of betrayal is often released from the devil to those closest to us. Our business partners, ministers, and friends can become targets of the devil when he wants to hinder what we are assigned to do.

Judas wasn't the enemy at first—he became vulnerable through unaddressed compromise.

If we do not disciple hearts well, even our most trusted allies can become vessels for sabotage.

When individuals become offended in the heart to the point of betrayal and treachery, they cause intentional harm on the leader and organization that they rise up against. As mature and emerging leaders, we have to understand the reality that we're targets for the devil and that he'd like to use us to afflict harm on the organization we're sworn to serve.

Leadership without spiritual warfare awareness is dangerous.

Every Kingdom assignment attracts both divine support and demonic resistance. Betrayal is one of the enemy's oldest weapons—but it is never greater than the grace to overcome.

Betrayal is one of the deepest wounds a leader can experience, especially when it comes from trusted companions and covenant relationships. In this opening chapter, we confront the spiritual weight and emotional cost of betrayal. Through the example of Judas and Jesus, we are reminded that betrayal is not only a relational rupture, but often a necessary part of divine assignment.

This chapter defines betrayal in covenant terms, explores its impact on organizational health, and emphasizes that leaders must remain postured—even when dishonor surrounds them.

Jesus' response to Judas teaches us that humility and integrity must never be abandoned, even in the presence of betrayal. Spiritual leaders are called to be discerning, vigilant, and forgiving, knowing that the enemy often uses those closest to us to carry out his schemes.

Betrayal does not have the final word. It may wound, but it cannot destroy what God has ordained—unless we let it.

Reflection & Review

Before closing this chapter, take a moment to reflect, release, and realign. These questions, statements, and prayers help you address betrayal through Scripture, whether you have hurt someone or been hurt. Let this be a sacred space for healing, forgiveness, and restoration.

Have you ever experienced betrayal while trying to build something meaningful—whether in ministry, family, or business?

_____

_____

_____

_____

_____

Have you taken the time to process that betrayal, or did you push past it and bury the pain?

_____

_____

_____

_____

Is there someone in your life that you may have unintentionally betrayed or walked away from prematurely?

_____

_____

_____

_____

What has betrayal taught you about yourself, your leadership, and your spiritual posture?

_____

_____

_____

_____

Are you open to healing in this area, or have you grown numb in order to survive?

_____

_____

_____

_____

Prayer of Mercy, Healing, and Forgiveness

"For it was not an enemy that reproached me; then I could have borne it: neither was it he that hated me that did magnify himself against me; then I would have hid myself from him: But it was thou, a man mine equal, my guide, and mine acquaintance. We took sweet counsel together, and walked unto the house of God in company."—Psalm 55:12–14 (KJV)

A prayer of surrender that releases pain and receives the wholeness of Christ.

This prayer invites you to release the sting of betrayal into God's hands and receive His mercy, healing, and strength to forgive.

—— Pray this Prayer ——

Heavenly Father, Your Word declares, "He healeth the broken in heart, and bindeth up their wounds" (Psalm 147:3). I come before You, acknowledging the pain that betrayal brings—but I also come trusting in Your ability to restore.

Lord, I cast this burden upon You, for Your Word says, "Cast thy burden upon the Lord, and He shall sustain thee" (Psalm 55:22). Where I have been wounded by someone I trusted, heal me. Where I have harbored bitterness or unforgiveness, cleanse me.

Father, Your Word says, "Create in me a clean heart, O God; and renew a right spirit within me" (Psalm 51:10). If I have ever been the cause of betrayal, knowingly or unknowingly, I ask for Your forgiveness. Let the blood of Jesus wash over my conscience.

Let's not betrayal define me, derail me, or divide me. You promised in Your Word, "No weapon that is formed against

thee shall prosper" (Isaiah 54:17), and I receive that even
betrayal will work for my good.

Today, I make room for Your mercy, both to receive and to
extend it. "Forgive us our debts, as we forgive our debtors"
(Matthew 6:12). I release those who have hurt me. I also repent
if I've ever become the Judas in someone else's story.

Now Father, I come boldly to the throne of grace, that I may
obtain mercy, and find grace to help in time of need (Hebrews
4:16). Heal me. Restore me. Keep me postured like Christ—
even in the face of betrayal. In Jesus' name, Amen.

Scripture for Meditation: The Lord is nigh unto them that are
of a broken heart; and saveth such as be of a contrite spirit." –
Psalm 34:18 (KJV)

Declarations & Decrees

"Thou shalt also decree a thing, and it shall be established unto thee..." Job 22:28 (KJV)

Decrees and Declarations
for the Betrayed and the Betrayer

"Thou shalt also decree a thing, and it shall be established
unto thee: and the light shall shine upon thy ways."
Job 22:28 (KJV)

This chapter exposed the weight of betrayal and the dangers of disconnection outside of God's timing. These decrees and declarations are crafted to help you renounce rebellion, embrace divine alignment, and declare your unwavering submission to the will of God.

—— **Decree & Declare** ——

I Decree and Declare: I decree that betrayal will not define my identity, delay my purpose, or destroy my posture.

No weapon that is formed against me shall prosper. Isaiah 54:17 (KJV)

I decree that I am healed from every soul wound caused by broken trust.

He healeth the broken in heart, and bindeth up their wounds." Psalm 147:3 (KJV)

I declare that my heart is clean, and I will lead without bitterness or revenge.

Create in me a clean heart, O God; and renew a right spirit within me." Psalm 51:10 (KJV)

I decree that I walk in the ministry of reconciliation and extend forgiveness as Christ forgave me.

And be ye kind one to another, tenderhearted, forgiving one another, even as God for Christ's sake hath forgiven you." Ephesians 4:32 (KJV)

What's Ahead…..

As you prepare to move into the next chapter, understand this: betrayal doesn't only come from outsiders. It most often comes through those we've welcomed into our inner circle.

In the next section, we'll look closely at the pain of betrayal through close relationships—where trust was once mutual, and loyalty was expected. Let's confront what happens when familiar voices become instruments of wounding.

"Proximity doesn't guarantee loyalty. Every leader must learn to discern hearts, not just hear words."

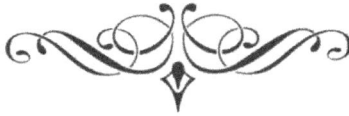

Chapter Two

Betrayal via Close Relationships

For it was not an enemy that reproached me; then I could have borne it... But it was thou, a man mine equal, my guide, and mine acquaintance. —**Psalm 55:12–13 (KJV)**

One of the most devastating realities in leadership is betrayal—not from an enemy, but from someone you've walked with in covenant. The grief of being wounded by a companion is a deep spiritual warfare that must be processed through the eyes of Christ.

Betrayal from within your circle is rarely about disagreement alone—it is often about misalignment, misunderstanding, or mismanagement of a spiritual connection.

David decried the treachery and betrayal of a friend who was closer than a brother. He cries out that it was his companion that he walked to the house of God with who exalted himself against him in betrayal.

- Psalm 55:12–13 (KJV) *For it was not an enemy that reproached me; then I could have borne it… But it was thou, a man mine equal, my guide, and mine acquaintance.*
- Psalm 55:14 (KJV) *We took sweet counsel together and walked unto the house of God in company.*

This wasn't a stranger. It was someone close. Someone in the circle. Unfortunately, the realm of betrayal and treachery often comes through close relationships.

David speaks further in Psalm 55:20–21: *He hath put forth his hands against such as be at peace with him: he hath broken his covenant." "The words of his mouth were smoother than butter, but war was in his heart: his words were softer than oil, yet were they drawn swords.*

David's attitude toward the betrayer is clear:

- He was formerly at peace with him.
- He was a covenant breaker.
- His words were smooth and soft.
- But war was in his heart.

Covenant is sacred. When someone breaks covenant, they don't just walk away from a person—they walk away from an assignment, a spiritual trust, and a divine alignment. Betrayal is not just an emotional experience—it's a spiritual breach.

David understood that this betrayal would not define him. He made a conscious decision:

Psalm 55:22 (KJV) *Cast thy burden upon the Lord, and He shall sustain thee: He shall never suffer the righteous to be moved.*

Betrayal must be cast, not carried. Carrying it contaminates your discernment. Casting it releases your soul to keep building.

As I've experienced betrayal, covenant breaking, and premature separation in ministry, I've come to recognize that not all betrayal is rooted in intentional harm. Some of it is willful, some unconscious, and some caught in a mixture of confusion and spiritual warfare.

Three States of Consciousness: Why People Betray

I believe Sigmund Freud's model of the three states of consciousness helps illustrate what occurs in moments of separation that are out of alignment with God's will and timing.

State of Consciousness	Human Will	God's Will Response
Conscious Mind	Informed Decisions	Willfully Defiant
Subconscious Mind	Uninformed Decisions	Rebellious or Emotionally Reactive
Unconscious Mind	Unaware Decisions	Lacking Discernment or Immaturity

These states can reveal how people interpret situations and make decisions—even decisions that result in betrayal.

Here's how I've seen it unfold:

Some people know the will of God but choose to disobey it. Others are emotionally led, making decisions without truly understanding the consequences. And some are simply unaware—operating from past wounds, pride, or spiritual blindness.

Regardless of how it happens, the result is often the same— damage to covenant relationships, delayed assignments, and leadership wounds.

As mature leaders, we must discern the origin of betrayal so we can respond in wisdom, not just pain.

Jesus showed us that sometimes betrayal is rooted in ignorance, not malice. This allows us to lead with compassion—even while holding the line of truth.

Luke 23:34 (KJV) *Father, forgive them; for they know not what they do.*

Whether you've been betrayed or have walked away from covenant relationships, this is the moment to release, forgive, and reset. Healing is not weakness—it's obedience.

Betrayal from afar is painful, but betrayal from those who've walked closely with you carries a weight that words often can't describe. This chapter explores the grief of being wounded by those who once shared covenant, counsel, and connection.

Like David, many leaders are left to process the shock that it wasn't an enemy—but a friend. Yet even in that pain, we are reminded to cast the burden upon the Lord and allow Him to sustain us.

I've also shared insight into the different states of consciousness that influence human behavior. Not all betrayal comes from outright rebellion—some comes from emotional immaturity, internal confusion, or spiritual blindness. Understanding this helps us release people to God, forgive deeply, and remain postured in love, even while healing.

Reflection & Review

Before we move into the questions for reflection, pause for a moment and allow the Holy Spirit to search your heart. Ministry and leadership are beautiful yet weighty assignments, and within them we often encounter both the joy of covenant relationships and the sting of betrayal.

Reflection is not meant to reopen wounds but to invite healing, growth, and restoration through Christ. These moments of honest review give God space to reveal where we've been hurt, where we may have unknowingly hurt others, and where He desires to carry burdens we were never meant to hold.

Have you ever been wounded by someone you walked closely with in ministry or leadership?

_____

_____

_____

_____

_____

_____

Did you allow yourself time to process the betrayal through the lens of Christ—or did you shut it down to survive?

_____

_____

_____

_____

Have you unknowingly wounded someone else due to offense, exhaustion, or internal pressure?

_____

_____

_____

_____

What burden are you carrying today that the Lord is asking you to cast upon Him?

_____

_____

_____

_____

Scripture for Meditation

Cast thy burden upon the Lord, and he shall sustain thee: he shall never suffer the righteous to be moved. —Psalm 55:22 (KJV)

Prayer for Healing and Realignment

"Cast thy burden upon the Lord, and he shall sustain thee: he shall never suffer the righteous to be moved."
Psalm 55:22 (KJV)

A prayer of surrender, healing, and restoration after betrayal.

When betrayal weighs heavy, the Lord invites us to exchange our burden for His sustaining strength. In His presence, we find healing and renewal.

—— Pray this Prayer ——

Heavenly Father, Your Word declares, "Cast thy burden upon the Lord, and He shall sustain thee: He shall never suffer the righteous to be moved" (Psalm 55:22).

Today I lay down the burden of betrayal. It was not an enemy that reproached me, but one who walked with me, prayed with me, and broke bread at my table (Psalm 55:12–14).

Heal me, O Lord, and I shall be healed; save me, and I shall be saved: for Thou art my praise (Jeremiah 17:14).

I choose to forgive, even as You have forgiven me (Colossians 3:13). Create in me a clean heart, O God, and renew a right spirit within me (Psalm 51:10).

I guard my heart with all diligence, for out of it flow the issues of life (Proverbs 4:23). Lord, teach me to walk in love, as Christ has loved me and given Himself for me (Ephesians 5:2).

Let integrity and uprightness preserve me, for I wait on Thee (Psalm 25:21). I will not be shaken. I will not retaliate. I will rise. In Jesus' name, amen.

Scripture for Meditation:

Psalm 55:22 (KJV): Cast thy burden upon the Lord, and He shall sustain thee: He shall never suffer the righteous to be moved.

Declarations & Decrees

"Thou shalt also decree a thing, and it shall be established unto thee..." Job 22:28 (KJV)

Decrees and Declarations for Betrayal in Close Relationships

These decrees and declarations are rooted in the authority of God's Word. Speak them boldly and consistently to realign your heart, break the spiritual residue of betrayal, and reaffirm your covenant with God.

As you declare truth over your life, your soul is reminded that you are not a victim of betrayal—you are a vessel of righteousness sustained by the Lord. Let each decree silence the voice of offense and re-establish your posture in purity, strength, and unwavering focus.

—— **Decree & Declare** ——

I decree that the pain of betrayal will not poison my purpose. Psalm 55:22

I decree that I will walk in spiritual discernment and not be deceived by flattering words. Proverbs 26:23

I declare that I will forgive those who were close to me and release the weight of the wound. Luke 23:34

I decree that God is restoring peace to every broken covenant I've cast upon Him. Isaiah 26:3

I decree that betrayal will not define me, for my identity is hidden in Christ. *Colossians 3:3*

I declare that no weapon formed against me shall prosper, and every tongue that rises against me in judgment is condemned. *Isaiah 54:17*

I decree that my heart will not be hardened by offense, but will remain tender before the Lord. *Ezekiel 36:26*

I declare that I am strong in the Lord and in the power of His might, and I will not be moved. *Ephesians 6:10*

I decree that the love of Christ is greater than the sting of betrayal, and His love governs my responses. *1 Corinthians 13:7*

I declare that God is vindicating me and setting my feet on a firm foundation. *Psalm 27:5–6*

I decree that I will guard my heart with diligence, and betrayal will not contaminate my future. *Proverbs 4:23*

I declare that God is turning what the enemy meant for evil into good for His glory. *Genesis 50:20*

I decree that I walk in the light, and darkness has no hold on me. *John 1:5*

I declare that integrity and righteousness preserve me as I wait upon the Lord. *Psalm 25:21*

What's Ahead....

In the next chapter, we will uncover the roots of betrayal—the internal and external influences that quietly open the door before the act ever takes place. Sometimes, the betrayal didn't start with their decision—it started with something they left unaddressed. Let's go deeper.

Unchecked wounds in the heart become open doors for betrayal. Guard your gates. Heal your places.

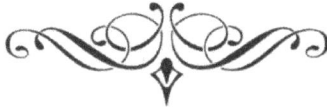

Chapter Three

Frequent Causes of Betrayal

"Can two walk together, except they be agreed?" —*Amos 3:3*
(KJV)

B etrayal rarely begins as an event. It begins as a seed. A thought left unchecked, a wound unhealed, or an offense unaddressed can fester into disconnection, rebellion, and eventual betrayal.

Before betrayal ever reaches the surface, it is nurtured quietly in the hidden spaces of the heart. When Lucifer betrayed God, it did not begin in the throne room—it began in his heart.

Ezekiel 28:17 says, *"Thine heart was lifted up because of thy beauty, thou hast corrupted thy wisdom by reason of thy brightness."* The corruption started internally. This is how betrayal operates: it works from the inside out.

As leaders, we must ask: what seeds are growing in us? What are we allowing to remain that God has called us to uproot? Seeds of comparison, offense, jealousy, entitlement, or ambition—if left unchecked—can become open doors to disloyalty.

Hebrews 12:15 warns us: *"Looking diligently lest any man fail of the grace of God; lest any root of bitterness springing up trouble you, and thereby many be defiled."* Seeds don't just affect the sower—they spread. If we don't confront the root, others may eat the fruit.

Even Judas didn't become a betrayer overnight. The compromise in Judas was present long before the kiss. The enemy simply watered what was already in place.

John 12:6 reveals, *"This he said, not that he cared for the poor; but because he was a thief, and had the bag, and bare what was put therein."*

If you are to remain pure in your call, you must discern and uproot the seeds of betrayal before they bloom. Ask the Lord to examine your heart.

Psalm 139:23 says, *"Search me, O God, and know my heart: try me, and know my thoughts."* The only safe heart is a surrendered one.

No one is above the possibility of betrayal—because no one is immune to temptation. But those who remain accountable, teachable, and surrendered will resist the subtle invitation to disconnect. We must remain rooted in humility and guarded against the weeds of pride.

These internal vulnerabilities open the door for deeper patterns. Let's explore five of the most frequent causes of betrayal and how they manifest.

Five Frequent Causes of Betrayal:

The cause of betrayal and treachery in the heart often begins with these five things:

Miscommunication

1 Corinthians 15:33–34 (KJV): "Be not deceived: evil communications corrupt good manners. Awake to righteousness, and sin not; for some have not the knowledge of God: I speak this to your shame."

Both sender and receiver must confirm effective communication. It is possible to feel like you have communicated clearly yet miss the mark. Likewise, it is easy to receive half the message and walk away with partial truth.

Miscommunication can birth offense and assumption, both of which nurture betrayal. Treacherous outcomes can be avoided through intentional communication and careful listening.

Illegal Voices

John 10:4–5 (KJV) "And when he putteth forth his own sheep, he goeth before them, and the sheep follow him: for they know his voice. And a stranger will they not follow, but will flee from him: for they know not the voice of strangers."

Genesis 3:1 (KJV) "Now the serpent was more subtil than any beast of the field which the Lord God had made. And he said unto the woman, Yea, hath God said..."

Illegal voices often masquerade as wisdom while carrying dishonorable motives. These voices may arise through people, ideologies, or even familiar spirits. The serpent gained Eve's ear, and deception was the outcome. Failing to discern and silence unauthorized voices can open doors to betrayal.

Impure Heart Motives

Proverbs 4:23 (KJV) *"Keep thy heart with all diligence; for out of it are the issues of life."*

The heart is the wellspring of action. Unchecked heart motives—such as selfish ambition, jealousy, or unresolved pain—become incubators for betrayal. Betrayal doesn't begin with an act; it begins with an intention. Unhealed trauma and impure desires can lead to broken covenants and damaged relationships. These wounds often require years of healing, counseling, and inner deliverance to fully overcome.

Imaginations

2 Corinthians 10:5 (KJV) *"Casting down imaginations, and every high thing that exalteth itself against the knowledge of God and bringing into captivity every thought to the obedience of Christ."*

The mind can be a battlefield. Those who betray often operate from false assumptions, personal offense, or misaligned perspectives. Imaginations—unreal conclusions—can masquerade as truth, leading people to separate prematurely from divine relationships and assignments. Scripture tells us to cast them down and subject every thought to Christ.

Offense
Proverbs 18:19 (KJV) *"A brother offended is harder to be won than a strong city: and their contentions are like the bars of a castle."*

Offense is a powerful wedge the enemy uses to divide relationships. Though sometimes separation is necessary (in cases of abuse or illegal conduct), offense without cause destroys unity. Reconciliation should always be our posture. Without it, offense festers into bitterness, which becomes fertile ground for betrayal.

Betrayal always begins as a seed in the hidden places of the heart. Left unguarded, those seeds—whether through miscommunication, illegal voices, impure motives, imaginations, or offense—grow into poisonous fruit that not only harms the one who carries them but also defiles many. The safeguard is a surrendered heart, searched by God and rooted in humility, accountability, and grace.

When we remain yielded, we are preserved from becoming betrayers and strengthened to withstand betrayal when it comes. With this foundation in place, we can now look more closely at how betrayal unfolds once it leaves the hidden place of the heart and shows itself in action.

Reflection & Review

The truths revealed in this chapter are not just for reflection—they are a call to personal inventory. Betrayal does not begin with action; it begins with access. As you walk through the following questions, declarations, and prayer, allow the Holy Spirit to expose any open doors in your heart.

These next moments are designed to realign your spirit, purify your motives, and guard your soul from subtle entrances the enemy uses to sow division. Let this time be a spiritual checkpoint as you contend for covenant integrity.

Have you ever acted on partial information and later regretted it?

_____

_____

_____

_____

_____

_____

_____

Can you recognize a time when an illegal voice led you into poor decisions?

_____

_____

_____

_____

_____

_____

_____

Have you confronted the motives of your heart before making major decisions?

_____

_____

_____

_____

_____

_____

_____

_____

Are you currently holding onto offense that could compromise your walk with God?

_____

_____

_____

_____

_____

_____

_____

Prayer for Guarding the Heart Against Betrayal

I come to You with a heart that longs to remain aligned with Your will. Search me, O God, and know my heart: try me and know my thoughts (Psalm 139:23).

A Prayer of Protection from Offense

*This prayer is rooted in the Word of God. Pray it sincerely,
allowing the Holy Spirit to examine and cleanse every hidden
area of your heart*

——Pray this Prayer——

Heavenly Father, If there be any root of bitterness, jealousy, or rebellion in me, I ask You to uproot it by Your Spirit. Help me to cast down imaginations and every high thing that exalts itself against Your knowledge (2 Corinthians 10:5).

Lord, let my heart remain guarded and diligent, for out of it flow the issues of life (Proverbs 4:23).

I reject the voice of the stranger and cling only to the voice of my Shepherd (John 10:4–5).

Cleanse my motives, purify my intentions, and help me to walk free of offense and unforgiveness. I decree that betrayal will not take root in me. In Jesus' name, amen.

Scripture for Meditation

"Keep thy heart with all diligence; for out of it are the issues of life." Proverbs 4:23 (KJV)

Declarations & Decrees

"Thou shalt also decree a thing, and it shall be established unto thee..." Job 22:28 (KJV)

Decrees and Declarations for a Guarded and Pure Heart

As you read these declarations aloud, speak them as weapons of truth to dismantle any hidden seeds of betrayal within you. Let your mouth align with God's Word to build guardrails around your heart.

——Decree & Declare ——

I decree that my heart is clean, my motives are pure, and my spirit is aligned with God's righteousness

Psalm 51:10 "Create in me a clean heart, O God; and renew a right spirit within me."

I declare that I will discern and reject every illegal voice attempting to speak into my destiny

John 10:5 *And a stranger will they not follow, but will flee from him: for they know not the voice of strangers."*

I decree that I cast down every vain imagination and bring every thought into captivity to the obedience of Christ

2 Corinthians 10:5 Casting down imaginations, and every high thing that exalteth itself against the knowledge of God and

bringing into captivity every thought to the obedience of Christ."

I declare that offense has no room in my heart—I walk in forgiveness, humility, and reconciliation

Proverbs 18:19 A brother offended is harder to be won than a strong city: and their contentions are like the bars of a castle."

What's Ahead...

As we examine the seeds and causes of betrayal, we must also take a deeper look at its fruit—disconnection, isolation, and the severing of God-ordained relationships.

In the next chapter, we'll explore how betrayal separates us from divine covenant and how to guard against disconnection before it fractures what God has joined.

"Covenant relationships are not sustained by comfort—they're sustained by commitment. Maturity stays when emotion wants to run."

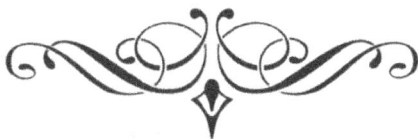

Chapter Four

Keys to Avoiding Betrayal

He that handleth a matter wisely shall find good: and whoso trusteth in the Lord, happy is he. —Proverbs 16:20 (KJV)

Betrayal is not only the result of offense or broken trust—it is often the byproduct of mismanaged relationships and spiritual immaturity.

In the Kingdom, we don't just protect ourselves from betrayal; we are called to steward our relationships with the wisdom of God so that betrayal is disarmed before it can manifest.

Just as David handled Saul with honor, even when Saul sought his life, we too must learn how to preserve covenant relationships and discern the timing, purpose, and boundaries of those assigned to our lives. Many betrayals are not rooted in evil intentions but in premature separations, poor communication, and unresolved personal wounds. As Kingdom builders, we must take responsibility for how we walk with others—especially in seasons of stretching and misunderstanding.

This chapter offers practical and spiritual wisdom for avoiding betrayal in your God-ordained connections. These are not merely suggestions but covenantal strategies that will protect your integrity, preserve divine relationships, and advance your maturity:

1. **Seek After and Yield to the Will of God in the Relationship:** When God assigns someone to your life, that relationship becomes a divine trust. You are not free to walk away based on discomfort. Many betrayals occur not out of rebellion, but impatience. True covenant will cost you something—comfort, convenience, and sometimes your opinion. The flesh will always seek escape from difficulty, but the Spirit leads us into endurance.

   Acts 17:26–27 (KJV) *...and hath determined the times before appointed, and the bounds of their habitation; That they should seek the Lord...*

Ecclesiastes 3:1 (KJV) *"To everything there is a season, and a time to every purpose under the heaven."*

When relationships are handled outside of God's timing, we often cause unnecessary pain to ourselves and others. Seek God's will and His timing in every relationship. Don't separate prematurely. Stay until the appointed release.

2. **Seek Understanding Before Drawing Conclusions:** One of the most dangerous assumptions in any relationship is that your perspective is complete. It is not. Understanding must be pursued with humility. The Word teaches us to incline our hearts toward wisdom and get understanding above all else.

3. **Proverbs 4:7 (KJV)** *Wisdom is the principal thing; therefore, get wisdom: and with all thy getting get understanding.*

Understanding is the lens through which we see truth more clearly. Without it, we may mislabel an ally as an enemy or misinterpret divine correction as rejection. This error can birth betrayal through misguided judgment. Before severing relationships or questioning someone's motives, labor to see through their lens.

Ask: What are they walking through that I don't see? What pain might be influencing their behavior? Wisdom gives grace, understanding guards the door of your heart.

4. **Pursue Peace—You Are a Minister of Reconciliation:**
   You were not just saved to go to Heaven—you were saved
   to be an agent of peace. The ministry of reconciliation is not
   for a select few; it is for every believer. When peace is
   pursued, offense loses power. When reconciliation is
   prioritized, betrayal becomes unnecessary.

   Hebrews 12:14–15 (KJV) Follow *peace with all men, and
   holiness, without which no man shall see the Lord...*

   2 Corinthians 5:18 (KJV) *And all things are of God, who
   hath reconciled us to himself by Jesus Christ, and hath given
   to us the ministry of reconciliation."*

Peace is not passive—it must be pursued. Sometimes, you must
initiate the conversation, humble yourself, and seek clarity even
when you were not at fault. The goal is not to win an argument,
but to win a brother.

5. **Give the Benefit of the Doubt:**

   Not every conflict is rooted in betrayal. Sometimes people are hurting, overwhelmed, or under demonic attack. Jesus taught us to respond not in vengeance but in mercy. This is a posture of maturity.

   Matthew 5:39–41 (KJV) *"...whosoever shall smite thee on thy right cheek, turn to him the other also... whosoever shall compel thee to go a mile, go with him twain."*

Giving others the benefit of the doubt means assuming the best until clarity proves otherwise. Betrayal often begins when we harden our hearts toward others because of unverified suspicion.

But love *believes all things, hopes all things* It doesn't rejoice in iniquity but in truth. (1 Corinthians 13:7).

Reflection & Review

In every relationship, timing, understanding, and grace are critical to maintaining alignment and avoiding betrayal. As you reflect, ask the Holy Spirit to uncover areas where impatience, misunderstanding, or offense may have disrupted divine connections.

These questions are crafted to help you realign with God's wisdom, preserve covenant relationships, and move forward with clarity and maturity.

Have I ever separated from a relationship prematurely because of pain, discomfort, or offense?

_____

_____

_____

_____

In what ways can I seek understanding before making assumptions about others' actions or motives?

_____

_____

_____

Have I truly embraced the ministry of reconciliation in my
daily relationships?

_____

_____

_____

_____

_____

_____

_____

How can I grow in extending mercy and giving others the
benefit of the doubt, especially when I feel wronged?

_____

_____

_____

_____

_____

_____

_____

Prayer for Honoring Divine Relationships

"To everything there is a season, and a time to every purpose under the heaven" (Ecclesiastes 3:1).

A Prayer of Wisdom, Patience, and Grace in God's Timing

This prayer helps you recognize the value of divine relationships and the importance of walking in wisdom, patience, and peace. It is an invitation to trust God's timing, extend grace, and remain faithful to the connections He has ordained.

——Pray this Prayer ——

Father, I thank You for the divine relationships You've placed in my life. Teach me to honor Your timing and trust Your will, even when I don't understand.

"To everything there is a season, and a time to every purpose under the heaven" (Ecclesiastes 3:1).

Help me walk in wisdom, for "wisdom is the principal thing" (Proverbs 4:7), and teach me to pursue peace with all people (Hebrews 12:14).
May my heart be a house of mercy.

I choose to turn the other cheek, walk the extra mile, and extend grace as You have done for me (Matthew 5:39–41).

Holy Spirit, give me discernment, patience, and humility. Deliver me from the urge to sever what You've assigned, and give me the strength to remain until Your timing releases me.

In Jesus' name, Amen.

Scripture for Meditation:

With all lowliness and meekness, with longsuffering, forbearing one another in love; Endeavouring to keep the unity of the spirit in the bond of peace. Ephesians 4:2–3 (KJV)

Declarations & Decrees

*"Thou shalt also decree a thing, and it shall be established
unto thee..." Job 22:28 (KJV)*

Decrees and Declarations
for the Betrayed and the Betrayer

"He that handleth a matter wisely shall find good: and whoso
trusteth in the Lord, happy is he."
Proverbs 16:20 (KJV)

Use these declarations as spiritual tools to align your heart with
the wisdom of God. Speak them aloud daily until they take root
in your mind, soul, and spirit. Decreeing truth out loud is a
spiritual strategy that empowers your walk and silences the lies
of offense, division, and assumption.

—— Decree and Declare ——

**I decree that I walk in the wisdom of God, and my steps in
relationships are ordered by Him.**

*He that handleth a matter wisely shall find good: and whoso
trusteth in the Lord, happy is he. Proverbs 16:20 (KJV)*

**I declare that I operate with understanding and see from the
lens of the Spirit, not the flesh.**

*Wisdom is the principal thing; therefore get wisdom: and with
all thy getting get understanding. Proverbs 4:7 (KJV)*

I decree that I am a minister of reconciliation, and peace is my portion in every relationship.

2 Corinthians 5:18 (KJV) And all things are of God, who hath reconciled us to himself by Jesus Christ, and hath given to us the ministry of reconciliation.

I declare that I give others the benefit of the doubt, walking in mercy, maturity, and grace.

Matthew 5:39–41 (KJV) But I say unto you, that ye resist not evil: but whosoever shall smite thee on thy right cheek, turn to him the other also. And if any man will sue thee at the law, and take away thy coat, let him have thy cloak also. And whosoever shall compel thee to go a mile, go with him twain.

Unforgiveness keeps you tied to betrayal. Forgiveness unlocks your future.

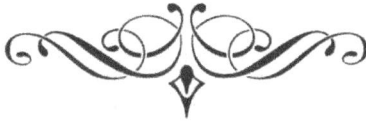

Chapter Five

Enduring the Pain of Betrayal

"Many are the afflictions of the righteous: but the Lord delivereth him out of them all."—Psalm 34:19 (KJV)

By now, through both Scripture and life experience, we recognize that betrayal and treachery are, tragically, common. These are not rare occurrences—they are part of the fallen condition of humanity. Whether in friendships, families, or the faith community, these wounds run deep. They pierce our trust and often leave lasting marks on the soul.

Even with our best intentions and utmost effort, we cannot fully avoid betrayal. We live in a world stained by sin, and as such, even those closest to us—those we love deeply—can become vessels of pain, sometimes unknowingly. Our response, as

Christ-followers, must be rooted in righteousness, mercy, and grace.

Our standard is not perfection, but reconciliation. For those who walk according to the Spirit, the ultimate aim is not just to endure betrayal, but to overcome it by reflecting the love of Christ. This requires supernatural grace. It requires choosing unity when division would be easier. It demands mending the breach when bitterness calls us to abandon the wall.

Jesus, in His final hours, prayed a profound prayer that still echoes today:

"That they all may be one; as thou, Father, art in me, and I in thee, that they also may be one in us..." —John 17:21 (KJV)

This oneness is not possible where betrayal is permitted to fester and fracture relationships. A divided Body cannot reflect a unified Christ. That's why the awareness of betrayal's effects is vital—because ignoring the pain only deepens the wound.

At times, betrayal flows from places outside our control. Family members, friends, or even spiritual leaders may operate from brokenness, trauma, or mental and emotional instability. When those we trust become instruments of harm, the wound can feel unbearable. But Jesus modeled the response that heals:

Father, forgive them; for they know not what they do. —Luke 23:34 (KJV)

This wasn't just a declaration from the cross—it was a spiritual strategy. Forgiveness liberates the offended more than the offender. It keeps us from being imprisoned by the actions of others.

When betrayal strikes, we must remember that our righteousness is not earned—it is imputed. Without Christ, even our best attempts at reconciliation are insufficient. As Isaiah reminds us:

But we are all as an unclean thing, and all our righteousnesses are as filthy rags…—Isaiah 64:6 (KJV)

This is why we look to our High Priest—Jesus—who not only sympathizes with our pain but endured the ultimate betrayal. His example assures us we are not alone:

Hebrews 4:15–16 (KJV) *For we have not an high priest which cannot be touched with the feeling of our infirmities; but was in all points tempted like as we are, yet without sin. Let us therefore come boldly unto the throne of grace, that we may obtain mercy, and find grace to help in time of need.*

Healing from betrayal begins at the throne. Grace flows from surrender. And strength comes when we fix our eyes on the One who endured betrayal for our redemption.

Betrayal is a reality that touches every believer at some point. While it cannot always be prevented, it can be endured with grace. This chapter reminds us that although betrayal wounds deeply, our response determines our healing.

Christ, who suffered the greatest betrayal, modeled forgiveness, unity, and mercy. Through His strength, we can overcome even the most painful breaches and remain anchored in righteousness, reconciliation, and spiritual maturity.

Reflection & Review

Betrayal, though painful, often reveals what's hidden deep within us. It tests our love, forgiveness, and willingness to walk in Christ's example. As you reflect on this chapter, allow the Holy Spirit to shine a light on any place in your heart that needs healing, release, or repentance. These questions are designed to help you pause, process, and position yourself for deeper reconciliation and inner restoration.

When have you experienced betrayal, and how did you respond emotionally and spiritually?

_____

_____

_____

Are there any unresolved offenses or breaches in your life that require forgiveness or reconciliation?

_____

_____

_____

_____

What practical steps can you take to keep your heart tender and free from bitterness?

_____

_____

_____

_____

_____

_____

_____

How has Jesus' response to betrayal challenged or encouraged you in your own journey?

_____

_____

_____

_____

_____

_____

_____

What's Ahead...

While wisdom helps us avoid many wounds, some betrayals still pierce deeply—often from those closest to us. The next chapter, "Enduring the Pain of Betrayal," will guide you through walking out forgiveness, releasing offense, and allowing God to heal the places where trust was broken.

Even when betrayal comes, grace can rebuild what pain tried to destroy. Prepare your heart to shift from guarding relationships to healing the heart.

Prayer of Forgiveness and Healing from Betrayal

"For if ye forgive men their trespasses, your heavenly Father will also forgive you. "Matthew 6:14 (KJV)

A Prayer of Mercy, Release, and Wholeness

This prayer is designed to help you release the pain of betrayal through forgiveness and embrace the healing that flows from Christ's mercy. As you pray, remember that forgiveness is not weakness—it is freedom that restores your heart and aligns you with the love of God.

——Pray this Prayer ——

Heavenly Father, I come boldly before Your throne of grace, that I may obtain mercy and find grace to help in my time of need (Hebrews 4:16).

Lord, I acknowledge the pain of betrayal and ask You to heal every wound. Just as Jesus said on the cross, "Father, forgive them; for they know not what they do" (Luke 23:34), I choose to forgive those who have hurt me.

I thank You that You are touched by the feeling of my infirmities and were in all points tempted as I am, yet without sin (Hebrews 4:15). Cleanse me, Lord, from bitterness and help me walk in forgiveness, just as Christ forgave me (Ephesians 4:32). I lay down every offense, every wound, and every unspoken pain.

Let love cover the multitude of sins (1 Peter 4:8), and let the peace of God rule in my heart (Colossians 3:15). I release those who hurt me and declare I am free, healed, and whole in Jesus' name. Amen.

Scripture Meditation:

And be ye kind one to another, tenderhearted, forgiving one another, even as God for Christ's sake hath forgiven you. — Ephesians 4:32 (KJV)

Declarations & Decrees

"Thou shalt also decree a thing, and it shall be established unto thee..." Job 22:28 (KJV)

Decrees and Declarations for a Clean Heart and a Strong Spirit

"So shall my word be that goeth forth out of my mouth: it shall not return unto me void, but it shall accomplish that which I please, and it shall prosper in the thing whereto I sent it."
Isaiah 55:11 (KJV)

Before declaring, take a moment to reflect on the truths from this chapter. Let your declarations flow from a heart postured in humility and strength, aligned with God's Word.

—— Declare & Decree ——

I decree that I am healed from every past betrayal and walk in the power of forgiveness.

But I say unto you, Love your enemies, bless them that curse you, do good to them that hate you, and pray for them which despitefully use you, and persecute you. —Matthew 5:44 (KJV)

I declare that the love of God flows through me, empowering me to forgive, restore, and reconcile.

And be ye kind one to another, tenderhearted, forgiving one another, even as God for Christ's sake hath forgiven you. — Ephesians 4:32 (KJV)

I decree that my heart remains clean and undefiled by bitterness or offense.

Let all bitterness, and wrath, and anger, and clamour, and evil speaking, be put away from you, with all malice. —Ephesians 4:31 (KJV)

I declare that I boldly approach the throne of grace and receive mercy and strength to endure.

Let us therefore come boldly unto the throne of grace, that we may obtain mercy, and find grace to help in time of need. Hebrews 4:16 (KJV)

Ministering to the Betrayed

Ministry to those who have experienced betrayal is both delicate and vital. As leaders and believers, we are often called to shepherd others through deep emotional and spiritual wounds. Betrayal leaves an imprint that, if not handled correctly, can fester into bitterness, mistrust, and spiritual stagnation. This bonus chapter serves as a guide for those ministering healing, restoration, and hope to the wounded.

Guiding Principles for Ministering to the Betrayed

1. Listen Without Judgment

Allow the person to share their story without interruption. Sometimes, the most healing thing we can do is give someone the gift of being heard.

Wherefore, my beloved brethren, let every man be swift to hear, slow to speak, slow to wrath (James 1:19, KJV).

2. Discern the Root Issue

Betrayal often opens the door to deeper wounds: rejection, abandonment, unworthiness. Ask the Holy Spirit for discernment to go beyond surface-level emotions and help the person identify and confront the root causes.

3. Bring the Word Gently

Ministering healing means applying truth with grace. Avoid using Scripture to pressure or shame. Instead, allow the Word to bring comfort and correction.

He sent His word, and healed them, and delivered them from their destructions. (Psalm 107:20, KJV).

4. Encourage Forgiveness, But Don't Force It

Forgiveness is a process. Lead them to the cross but be patient as they navigate their emotions. Emphasize that forgiveness sets them free.

And be ye kind one to another, tenderhearted, forgiving one another, even as God for Christ's sake hath forgiven you (Ephesians 4:32, KJV).

5. Pray Strategically

Target strongholds of rejection, bitterness, anger, and fear in prayer. Encourage the betrayed to pray over their own soul and invite the Holy Spirit to bring deep healing.

6. Create a Safe Environment

Whether in counseling, small group, or altar ministry, those healing from betrayal need safety and confidentiality. Honor their story. Do not rush their healing timeline.

7. Point Them Toward Community

Isolation is often a byproduct of betrayal. Help them rebuild trust in healthy relationships. Invite them into community that nurtures and restores.

8. Affirm Their Identity in Christ

Remind them that they are not what happened to them. They are who God says they are. Lead them through affirmations and Scriptures that rebuild self-worth and confidence in the Father's love.

9. Follow Up

Healing is not a one-time encounter. Create opportunities for ongoing support. Check in, offer resources, and be available.

10. Minister From a Healed Place

Make sure your own heart is free from offense, bitterness, or unresolved betrayal. Ministering from a wounded place can transfer pain instead of healing.

Create in me a clean heart, O God; and renew a right spirit within me" (Psalm 51:10, KJV).

Affirmations of Renewal

These affirmations are designed to help you renew your mind and align your heart with God's truth. Speak them aloud daily, especially when feelings of hurt, rejection, or confusion arise. Let the Word of God reframe your identity and restore your confidence.

1. I am not defined by the pain of my past. I am renewed by the grace of Christ. (2 Corinthians 5:17)

2. I release all bitterness, resentment, and anger. I walk in the freedom of forgiveness. (Ephesians 4:31-32)

3. I am accepted in the beloved. I am chosen and dearly loved by God. (Ephesians 1:6; Colossians 3:12)

4. I have the mind of Christ. I will not be led by vain imaginations or emotional confusion. (1 Corinthians 2:16; 2 Corinthians 10:5)

5. I am surrounded by God's favor like a shield. Betrayal will not define my future. (Psalm 5:12)

6. I will not fear being hurt again. Perfect love casts out fear. (1 John 4:18)

7. I am healed by the stripes of Jesus. My soul is being restored daily. (Isaiah 53:5; Psalm 23:3)

8. God is the restorer of my broken places. He makes all things new. (Isaiah 61:3; Revelation 21:5)

9. I am strong in the Lord and in the power of His might. I am not defeated. (Ephesians 6:10)

10. My heart is guarded by the peace of God. I will not be moved by chaos or betrayal. (Philippians 4:7)

11. I am led by the Spirit of God. I will no longer be influenced by illegal voices. (Romans 8:14; John 10:5)

12. I forgive those who hurt me, and I bless those who cursed me. I am free. (Luke 6:28; Matthew 5:44)

13. God is writing a new story with my life. My testimony will bring others healing. (Revelation 12:11)

14. I belong to the Kingdom of God. I am not an orphan or abandoned. (Romans 8:15-16)

15. I am advancing with purpose, clarity, and Kingdom alignment. (Proverbs 3:5-6; Matthew 6:33)

Repeat these daily until they become the loudest voice in your spirit. Let God's truth anchor your identity, and may your healing become a testimony of His power and grace.

Walking Forward in Wholeness

Betrayal, while deeply painful, does not have the final word. From Genesis to Revelation, the Bible chronicles moments of heartbreak and human failure—and yet we see God's redemptive hand always making a way for restoration. If you've walked through betrayal, or even if you've been the betrayer, there is still hope for healing.

We serve a Savior who was betrayed, rejected, and wounded, yet still offered forgiveness, reconciliation, and love. As believers, we are called to walk the same path—not by our own strength, but through the power of the Holy Spirit.

Let this book serve as a mirror to examine your own heart, a compass to realign your relationships, and a healing balm to wounds you may still carry. If you've been carrying the weight of offense, guilt, or broken trust, release it today at the feet of Jesus. Allow Him to do the deep work. He restores the soul.

May the grace of God empower you to walk in humility, discernment, forgiveness, and unwavering love. May you guard your heart with diligence, keep your spirit aligned with righteousness, and lean into the ministry of reconciliation. There is life after betrayal, and there is purpose beyond the pain.

You are not alone. You are not disqualified. You are being refined.

And as you continue your journey, may your heart remain clean, your hands stay pure, and your eyes fixed on the One who is Faithful and True.

Blessings,

Apostle Kenneth E. Toney

Additional Prayers & Scriptures

In times of betrayal, the heart is often left wounded and the spirit heavy with grief. Yet, God has given us His Word and prayer as the pathway to healing, restoration, and renewed strength.

These additional prayers, paired with scriptural references, serve as anchors for the soul—reminding us that forgiveness, blessing, love, and reconciliation are not burdens but Kingdom responses that align us with the heart of the Father.

As you meditate on these prayers and scriptures, allow the Holy Spirit to search your heart, release the weight of offense, and lead you into freedom, peace, and wholeness through Christ.

Forgiveness

Father, I choose to forgive those that have hurt me through acts of betrayal, the breaking of mutually agreed covenants, failure to meet agreed upon expectations, breaching of relationships unilaterally, violating mutual trust and those that have willfully left the relationship with malice, gossip and slander.

"For if ye forgive men their trespasses, your heavenly Father will also forgive you." Matthew 6:14 (KJV)

Blessings

I choose to bless those that have cursed me and to pray blessings, peace and purpose upon those who have wished me harm in breaching the relationship. I choose to forgive every individual that has betrayed me willfully or unintentionally in any shape, form or fashion. I further declare that all collateral damage done to others, harm to the Body of Christ and to innocent individuals by the breach be covered in the blood of Jesus and sealed by his daily release of mercy.

"Bless them which persecute you: bless, and curse not." Romans 12:14 (KJV)

Love

I choose the pathway of love, forgiveness and repentance for my part in any betrayal, unmet expectations, violation of mutual trust and breach in the Body of Christ that came about by my own actions, known and unknown. I further repent for any negative or carnal emotions or fleshly reaction to the betray, breach or violation of trust. I choose to walk in love and to employ the fruit of Holy Spirit at all times and on all occasions.

"And above all things have fervent charity among yourselves: for charity shall cover the multitude of sins." 1 Peter 4:8 (KJV)

Reconciliation

According to the will of the Father and demonstrated repentance and forgiveness concerning each act of betrayal, I am open to reconciliation with those who perpetrated the breach and those affected by the fallout. I choose to do my part in offering and responding to attempts at reconciliation and restoration of the relationship according to the will of the Father.

"And all things are of God, who hath reconciled us to himself by Jesus Christ, and hath given to us the ministry of reconciliation." 2 Corinthians 5:18 (KJV)

Choose to Demonstrate the Fruit of the Spirit in the Face of Betrayal

Galatians 5:10-17 (KJV) : I have confidence in you through the Lord, that ye will be none otherwise minded: but he that troubleth you shall bear his judgment, whosoever he be. And I, brethren, if I yet preach circumcision, why do I yet suffer persecution? then is the offence of the cross ceased. I would they were even cut off which trouble you. For, brethren, ye have been called unto liberty; only use not liberty for an occasion to the flesh, but by love serve one another.

For all the law is fulfilled in one word, even in this; Thou shalt love thy neighbour as thyself. But if ye bite and devour one another, take heed that ye be not consumed one of another. This I say then, Walk in the Spirit, and ye shall not fulfil the lust of the flesh. For the flesh lusteth against the Spirit, and the Spirit against the flesh: and these are contrary the one to the other: so that ye cannot do the things that ye would.

Choose to be Reconciled

Matthew 5:23-25 (KJV)

Therefore if thou bring thy gift to the altar, and there remberest that thy brother hath ought against thee; Leave there thy gift before the altar, and go thy way; first be reconciled to thy brother, and then come and offer thy gift. Agree with thine adversary quickly, whiles thou art in the way with him; lest at any time the adversary deliver thee to the judge, and the judge deliver thee to the officer, and thou be cast into prison.

Choose to Overcome Offence

Matthew 18:6-11 (KJV)

But whoso shall offend one of these little ones which believe in me, it were better for him that a millstone were hanged about his neck, and that he were drowned in the depth of the sea. Woe unto the world because of offences! for it must needs be that offences come; but woe to that man by whom the offence cometh!

Wherefore if thy hand or thy foot offend thee, cut them off, and cast them from thee: it is better for thee to enter into life halt or maimed, rather than having two hands or two feet to be cast into everlasting fire. And if thine eye offend thee, pluck it out, and cast it from thee: it is better for thee to enter into life with one eye, rather than having two eyes to be cast into hell fire. Take heed that ye despise not one of these little ones; for I say unto you, That in heaven their angels do always behold the face of my Father which is in heaven. For the Son of man is come to save that which was lost.

Choose to Forgive and Attempt to Reconcile
Matthew 18:15-17 (KJV)

Moreover if thy brother shall trespass against thee, go and tell him his fault between thee and him alone: if he shall hear thee, thou hast gained thy brother. But if he will not hear thee, then take with thee one or two more, that in the mouth of two or three witnesses every word may be established. And if he shall neglect to hear them, tell it unto the church: but if he neglect to hear the church, let him be unto thee as an heathen man and a publican.

Demonstrate Reconciliation *versus* Separation
2 Corinthians 5:18-20 (KJV)

And all things are of God, who hath reconciled us to himself by Jesus Christ, and hath given to us the ministry of reconciliation; To wit, that God was in Christ, reconciling the world unto himself, not imputing their trespasses unto them; and hath committed unto us the word of reconciliation. Now then we are ambassadors for Christ, as though God did beseech you by us: we pray you in Christ's stead, be ye reconciled to God.

Choose to walk in love

Galatians 5:22-26 (KJV)

But the fruit of the Spirit is love, joy, peace, longsuffering, gentleness, goodness, faith, meekness, temperance: against such there is no law. And they that are Christ's have crucified the flesh with the affections and lusts. If we live in the Spirit, let us also walk in the Spirit. Let us not be desirous of vain glory, provoking one another, envying one *another.*

ABOUT THE AUTHOR

Apostle Kenneth E. Toney
Apostolic Leader, Visionary, and Servant of the Nations
Founder & Senior Pastor
Dwelling Place International Church

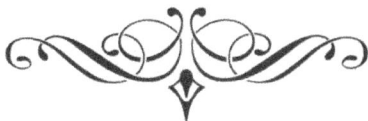

Apostle Kenneth E. Toney

Apostle Ken Toney has faithfully served as the Senior Pastor of Dwelling Place International Church in Collierville, Tennessee, alongside his wife, Pastor Carolyn Toney, for more than 15 years. Together, they have built a thriving ministry marked by vision, integrity, and a heart for the nations.

Apostle Ken carries a strong apostolic mandate for Leadership Development, Church Planting, and Strategic Intercession. His passion for missions and evangelism has taken him across the nation and into the nations, where he proclaims the Gospel message of hope, faith, and Kingdom transformation. Known for his generous spirit, deep compassion, and unwavering commitment to truth, he provides wise and steady guidance to his congregation and beyond.

Under his leadership, Dwelling Place International Church has flourished with a clear mission to Gather Believers, Engage and Equip Disciples, and Send Leaders into Destiny. Beyond the local church, Apostle Ken also serves as President of City Dwellers, Inc., a non-profit organization dedicated to Grocery Relief, Disaster Response, and Urban Development. He and Pastor Carolyn actively support global missions, with ongoing works in Accra, Ghana; Merida, Mexico; and Bangalore, India.

Their 26-year marriage stands as a testimony of love and faithfulness, and together they are the proud parents of Kennedie (24) and Timothy (19). In addition to their ministry assignments, Apostle Ken continues to walk in his marketplace calling as an IT Manager, while Pastor Carolyn serves as a licensed Cosmetology Instructor and Educator with MSCS. Both remain committed to lifelong learning, pursuing ongoing training and certifications through various ministry schools and biblical institutes.

References

1. Boag, S. (n.d.). *Conscious, Preconscious, and Unconscious*. In *Encyclopedia of Personality and Individual Differences*.

2. Bargh, J. A. (2013). Our unconscious mind. *Scientific American*, *310*(1), 30-37. https://doi.org/10.1038/scientificamerican0114-30

3. Zimmermann, J., Löffler-Stastka, H., Huber, D., et al. (2015). Is it all about the higher dose? Why psychoanalytic therapy is an effective treatment for major depression. *Clinical Psychology & Psychotherapy*, *22*(6), 469-487. https://doi.org/10.1002/cpp.1917

www.ingramcontent.com/pod-product-compliance
Lightning Source LLC
Chambersburg PA
CBHW052214270326
41931CB00011B/2352